RECLAIMING OUR LIVES

FROM STRESS

PAMELA WAKEFIELD

Reclaiming Our Lives from Stress

Disclaimer:

Note: This workbook contains the opinions and ideas of its author. It is intended to provide informational material about the subject matter and is not a medical publication. The information provided is not intended to substitute for or replace medical or professional treatment. If you are in need of medical or professional help, please consult your provider.

Printed in the United States of America

TABLE OF CONTENTS

My Story

I wrote Reclaiming Our Lives from Stress as a guide to help women identify stressful living. I wanted women to be informed, especially mothers, about the dangers of stressful living, how stress affects the mind and body and ways to relieve stress.

The turning point in my life began in 1997 when I became ill and there was no diagnosis or treatment to the symptoms that were being manifested in my body. During that year, my life consisted of regular emergency visits, ongoing doctor appointments, visits to specialists, and expensive medical bills. I was given many diagnoses such as Hiatal Hernia, GERD, Fibromyalgia, IBS, Skin Disorders, Diverticulitis, Anxiety, Panic Attacks, Depression, Migraines, Reflux, Fatigue, and Nerve Pain.

After months and years of suffering in silence, the root cause to every diagnosis was related to STRESS!

Note to READER

- This information contained in this workbook is for awareness and educational purposes. This workbook is not intended to treat, diagnose, or cure any medical condition nor serve as medical advice.

- This workbook has five main objectives that the reader will learn:

  - **THE DEFINITION OF STRESS**

  - **HOW STRESS AFFECTS THE MIND AND BODY**

  - **THE PHYSICAL AND MENTAL SIGNS OF STRESS**

  - **TIPS ON RELIEVING STRESS**

  - **IMPLEMENTING A STRESS RELIEF PLAN**

FACTS!

- Many times, women especially mothers are faced with stressful conditions due to the many roles we are given. We often vocalize how stressed we are but are unaware of the dangers of how too much stress can affect our physical and mental health.

- Throughout history, Black women have been identified as being strong and resilient and having the ability to adapt to difficult and stressful situations. But the bad news, is that many of us could be in danger of developing stress-related illnesses, because of too much stress. Often times we lack the balance we need and find ourselves taking care of everyone else and putting our needs last.

- There appears to be a false perception that Black women can handle everything, without there being any repercussions to our health and well-being. Stressful living for long periods of times can have damaging effects on our health. It can also lead one to feeling depleted, overwhelmed, unbalanced, and ill. Sometimes the effects of stressful living can also leave us feeling unappreciated, unwanted, disrespected, unloved, bitter, angry, and/or depressed.

- Stress is not easily talked about or even understood in our circles, because stress is perceived as a weakness. It's pressed upon us to be quiet, don't complain, be strong, and keep going. But what about the times when you feel like you can't go on anymore? What do you do? To whom do you turn, and who can you trust? Unfortunately, in many cases, we suffer in silence.

- I'm not sure what keeps us going, when we are mentally, physically, and emotionally worn out. I don't know if these behaviors are learned, culturally influenced, or whether it's something innately driving us. Whatever it is, we must make our health and well-being a priority by identifying stressful events and learn ways to relieve stress and have balance.

- In my previous book, *Reclaiming My Life from Stress: A Black Mother's Journey from Stressful Living*, I informed and shared with women on how stress affected my physical and mental well-being and how I had to take the steps to reclaim my life. *Reclaiming Our Lives from Stress* workbook provides tips and a plan to help women reclaim their life from stress too.

My heart's desire is for women to be informed and aware of the dangers of too much stress, so that you will be empowered to live a health, peaceful and stress-free lifestyle.

Peace and Blessings,

Pamela

TAKE THE STRESS QUIZ #1

STRESS IS AVOIDABLE?

STRESS CAN CAUSE WEIGHT LOSS?

Yes Or No?

TOO MUCH STRESS CAN CAUSE BELLY FAT?

STRESS IS EASILY DIAGNOSED?

TAKE THE STRESS QUIZ #2

60% OF DOCTOR'S VISITS ARE STRESS-RELATED

ALL STRESS IS BAD

True or False?

STRESS CAN BE LINKED TO ANXIETY OR DEPRESSION

CHRONIC STRESS CAN STRENGTHEN YOUR IMMUNE SYSTEM

The answers to this questionnaire can be found in the back of the book.

WHAT IS STRESS?

1. THE NERVOUS SYSTEM'S RESPONSE TO THE EXTERNAL AND INTERNAL IRRITANTS (PRESSURES)

2. THE RATE OF WEAR AND TEAR ON THE MIND AND BODY

3. A PERSON'S INABILITY TO COPE WITH THE PRESSURE AND DEMANDS

4. REACTION TO A PHYSICAL, MENTAL, OR EMOTIONAL STIMULUS THAT UPSETS THE BODY'S NATURAL BALANCE

You may be asking yourself, what is stress, what's the big deal and how can stress negatively affect my health? Give me a few minutes and I'll explain.

You may hear people say it's normal to experience stress in small doses because it gives us the burst of energy we need to complete a task. However, stress becomes a problem when we experience too much of it. Stress that we experience for long periods of time can weaken our immune system, increase our blood pressure, affect our heart, put us at risk for anxiety and/or depression and can leave us feeling fatigue and much more.

Stress is real, and each person perceives and responds to stress differently. Stress is defined as the nervous system's response to external and internal irritants that affect the mind and body and the inability to cope with life demands. When a person experiences stress for long periods of time (also known as chronic stress) it puts an individual at risk for developing stress-related illnesses which can affect a person's physical and mental health.

Being overly stressed can negatively affect your health and impact your life. Researchers indicate that 75 to 85 % of physician visits are stress-related and that chronic stress weakens the immune system and makes one susceptible to illness and disease. Stress can affect the nervous, endocrine, cardiovascular, digestive, respiratory systems, and more.

Not all stress is caused by external factors. Stress can also be internal or self-generated, which is emotional stress. This can occur when someone worries excessively or have negative, pessimistic or irrational thoughts about something that may or may not happen. Having anger, resentment, low self-esteem, bitterness, grief, guilt and experiencing a traumatic event can also negatively affect your emotions.

All stress is not considered bad. there is good stress, such as: the birth of a new baby, job promotion, going back to school, purchasing a new home, starting a business, changing a career, getting married, and etc. All of these events are good, but they can be stressful too, because they will require adjustments and/or additional responsibilities.

However, in time the demands will eventually balance out, especially if you learn how to pace yourself and adjust to the newness that's been added to your life.

There are different types of stress. For example, there is short-term stress or situational stress. This occurs when you may be feeling pressured, anxious or overwhelmed about an event or situation that is happening in the moment. Such as: waiting in a long line, a traffic jam, working on a project or taking a test. The stressful event occurs and then it's over. Your body responses will return to its normal state and you will no longer feel anxious about the event, because the event is over. I want you to understand situational stressful events cannot always be avoided, such as waiting in a traffic jam or long grocery line, but how you respond to the stressful event can make a difference.

There is another stress I want to talk about and that is called <u>chronic stress</u>. This type of stress is considered negative and can be harmful. This type of stress can become a problem and affect your health when you experience prolonged stress or constant stress for weeks, months or even years.

Chronic stress is defined as a prolonged and constant feeling of stress that can negatively affect your health if it goes untreated. It can be caused by the everyday pressures of family and work or by traumatic situations (Verywellmind.org). It's the response to emotional pressure suffered for a prolonged period of time in which an individual

perceives they have little or no control. (Wikipedia).
Examples of this type of stress are work-related
stress, financial stress, unhealthy relationships,
divorce, loss of home, car or job, health problems,
parenting, caring for a loved one and etc.

Chronic stress has been linked to heart disease,
cancer, obesity, depression, anxiety disorders, heart
attacks, digestive problems, autoimmune disorders,
skin conditions, and much more. It can also affect
concentration and memory.

When a person experiences a stressful event the
brain releases hormones into the bloodstream called
cortisol and epinephrine (also known as adrenaline).
It's been noted that too much epinephrine can be
harmful to your heart and can affect how cells are

able to regenerate. Epinephrine is a hormone secreted by the adrenal glands, especially in conditions of stress. Stress is your body's way of responding to any kind of demand or threat. (helpguide.com).

THE FIGHT OR FLIGHT RESPONSE!

WHAT HAPPENS TO THE BODY WHEN YOU EXPERIENCE STRESS?

FIGHT OR FLIGHT RESPONSE

- Heart Beats Faster
- Blood Pressure Increases
- Blood Clots
- Nausea
- Muscle Tension
- Slowed digestion
- Rise in cholesterol

To get a better picture of how stress affects the mind and body, I want you to imagine walking in the park and seeing a pit bull running towards you. Immediately, your response will be either to fight the pit bull or to run for cover. This is called the *fight-or-flight response*. The body and mind know there is danger ahead and begins to prepare itself to *fight or take flight*. This is the same response that your body would encounter during a stressful event.

The *fight-or-flight* response is a physiological one that affects your nervous system. It occurs in response to a perceived harmful event, attack, or threat to survival. This response will start alarming your body to respond to the event. The body was made to prepare itself to perform during a time like this. It starts with the hypothalamus in your brain, and then a combination of hormones and nerves will prompt your adrenal glands to release adrenaline and cortisol. Adrenaline increases your heart rate and blood pressure, and cortisol suppresses the digestive system and affects the immune system. This response affects your mood as well.

Your heart will beat faster, blood pressure will increase, you may have stomach pain, your blood will begin to start clotting, you may feel cold or nausea, you may feel tension in your neck, your digestion will slow up or stop, cholesterol levels rise. You may become irritable, frightened, out of control, edgy, or nervous, but when the stressful event is over, your body will return to its normal state.

However, the problem occurs when an individual suffers with constant stress and the mind and body stays in a heightened state. The body will respond to stressful events as if one is in danger of being attacked. The body doesn't know how to distinguish between a stressful event or a perceived threat or danger.

The body was created to prepare us for a dangerous event so that we have the capabilities and energy to respond to the situation, but the body was not designed for one to experience continuous stress and demands for long periods of time. This type of pressure or consistent overload is damaging to one's physical and mental health.

In 1967, psychiatrists Thomas Holmes and Richard Rahe conducted a study and developed a stress scale to determine if stress is contributed to illness. The Holmes and Rahe Stress Scale have been used to determine the amount of stress one experience within a year and to rate the person's score. The scale suggests the higher the score, the more likely the person is to become ill.

Please see the Holmes and Rahe Stress Scale that's listed on pages 28-30 of this book or you can search on the Internet.

TYPES OF STRESS

SITUATIONAL

Short term worry or concern that can cause physical symptoms. But once the situation has ended the stress leaves.

CHRONIC

Occurs when demands seem to not have an end and there is no solution. There is constant wear and tear on the mind and body.

GOOD

Occurs when a positive event causes a feeling of excitement and there is no threat or fear.

EMOTIONAL

Involves the experience of negative affects such as anxiety, depression, anger, grief, guilt, low self esteem and traumatic events

DID YOU KNOW!

✓ Too much stress can upset your natural balance and can possibly affect your health

✓ No one can define stress for you, only you know what causes you to be stressed

✓ Stress can affect your physical and mental well-being

✓ Stress affects your mood and can cause you to be short tempered or inpatient with others

✓ Stress can make you feel unbalanced and overwhelmed

✓ Chronic stress has been linked to anxiety, depression, and other illnesses and diseases

- ✓ Negative emotions such as fear, worry, grief and anger releases stress hormones

- ✓ Stress is not always easily diagnosed

- ✓ Stress is not always easily understood

- ✓ Stress can affect your relationships

HOW STRESS AFFECTS THE MIND AND BODY

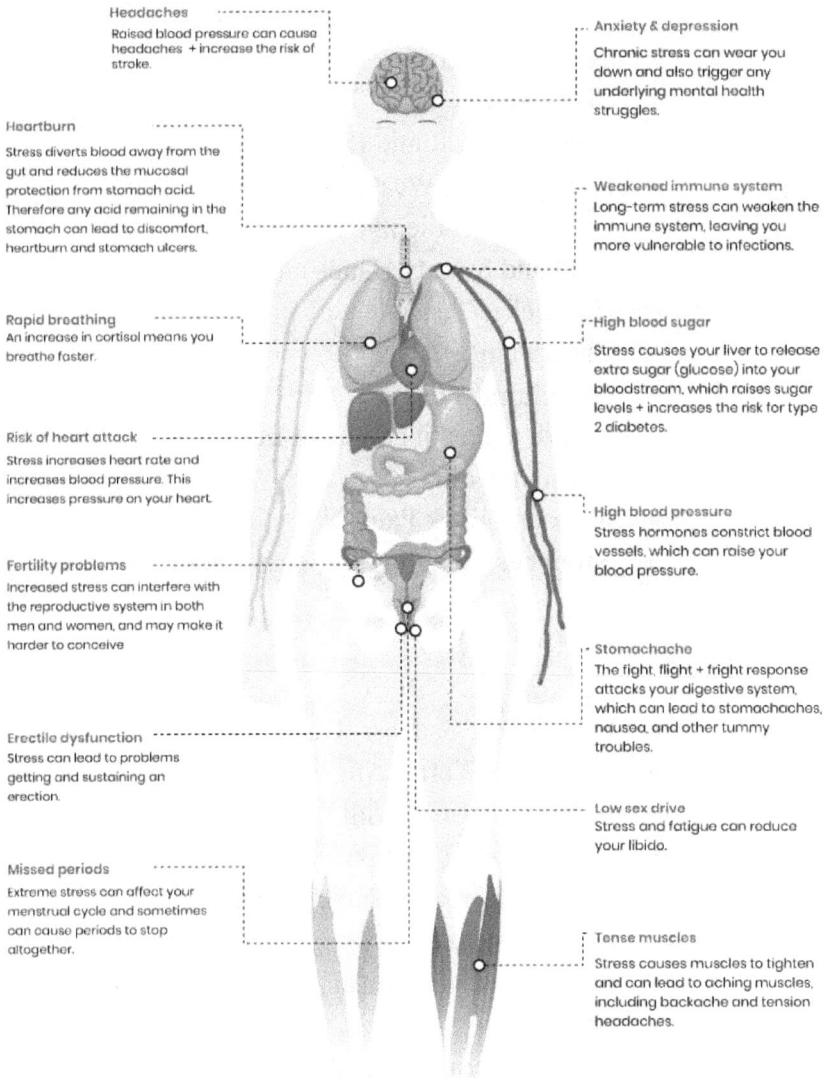

Headaches
Raised blood pressure can cause headaches + increase the risk of stroke.

Anxiety & depression
Chronic stress can wear you down and also trigger any underlying mental health struggles.

Heartburn
Stress diverts blood away from the gut and reduces the mucosal protection from stomach acid. Therefore any acid remaining in the stomach can lead to discomfort, heartburn and stomach ulcers.

Weakened immune system
Long-term stress can weaken the immune system, leaving you more vulnerable to infections.

Rapid breathing
An increase in cortisol means you breathe faster.

High blood sugar
Stress causes your liver to release extra sugar (glucose) into your bloodstream, which raises sugar levels + increases the risk for type 2 diabetes.

Risk of heart attack
Stress increases heart rate and increases blood pressure. This increases pressure on your heart.

High blood pressure
Stress hormones constrict blood vessels, which can raise your blood pressure.

Fertility problems
Increased stress can interfere with the reproductive system in both men and women, and may make it harder to conceive

Stomachache
The fight, flight + fright response attacks your digestive system, which can lead to stomachaches, nausea, and other tummy troubles.

Erectile dysfunction
Stress can lead to problems getting and sustaining an erection.

Low sex drive
Stress and fatigue can reduce your libido.

Missed periods
Extreme stress can affect your menstrual cycle and sometimes can cause periods to stop altogether.

Tense muscles
Stress causes muscles to tighten and can lead to aching muscles, including backache and tension headaches.

INDICATORS OF FEELING STRESSED

PHYSICAL (BODY)

- Tensed Muscles
- Body Aches
- Rapid Pulse, Rapid Breathing
- Fatigue/Tired/Weakness
- Digestive Problems
- Cold and Sweaty Hands and Feet
- Headaches/Tension
- Chest Pain
- Overeating/Weight Gain/Undereating/Weight Loss
- Constant Colds
- Neck and Back Pain
- Numbness/Tingling in Extremities

MENTAL (MIND)

- Depression, Sadness, Unhappiness
- Excessive Worry, Anger, Frustration, Fear
- Inability to Cope with Life Demands
- Withdrawal, Isolation
- Anxious/Anxiety, Panic Attacks
- Nervousness
- Irritable/Mood Swings
- Forgetfulness
- Can't sleep/Insomnia/Too much sleep

- Inability in Making Decisions
- Loss of Interest to do things
- Defensive
- Angry
- And more....

Please note the above indicators are just a few of the signs that someone may experience if they are constantly stressed. Each person responds to stress differently. This list is not to diagnosis or treat any medical or mental condition, but to provide information on the effects of stress.

Disclaimer: Please seek medical and/or professional help if needed.

The Holmes-Rahe Life Stress Inventory

This scale was designed to determine the chances an individual developing a stress related illness based on life events that occurred within a year. .Mark down the point value of each of these life events that has happened to you in one year and total the points

Death of a spouse	100
Divorce	75
Marital separation from mate	65
Detention in jail or institution	63
Death of a close family member	63
Major personal injury or illness	53
Marriage	50
Being fired at work	47
Martial reconciliation with mate	45
Retirement from work	45
Major change in the health or behavior of a family member	44
Pregnancy	40
Sexual difficulties	39
Gaining a new family member	39
(i.e., birth, adoption, older adult moving in, etc.)	
Major business adjustment	39
Major change in financial state	38
(i.e., a lot worse or better off than usual)	
Death of a close friend	37
Changing to a different line of work	36
Major change in # of arguments w/spouse	35
Taking on a mortgage	31

Foreclosure on a mortgage or loan	30
Major change in responsibilities at work	29
Son or daughter leaving home	29
In-law troubles	29
Outstanding personal achievement	28
Spouse beginning or ceasing work	26
Beginning or ceasing formal schooling	26
Major change in living condition (new home, remodeling, deterioration of neighborhood or home, etc.)	25
Revision of personal habits (dress manners, associations, quitting smoking	24
Trouble with boss	23
Major changes in working hours/conditions	20
Changes in residence	20
Changing to a new school	20
Major change in usual type and/or amount of recreation	19
Major change in church activity	19
Major change ins social activities (clubs, movies, visiting)	18
Taking on a loan (car, tv, freezer, etc.)	17
Major change in sleeping habits (a lot more or a lot less)	16
Major change in number of family get-togethers	15
Major change in eating habits	15
Vacation	13
Major holidays	12
Minor violations of the law (traffic tickets, jaywalking, disturbing the peace, etc.)	11
(Add up all the points to find your score) TOTAL	_____

150 points or less means a relatively low amount of life change and a low susceptibility to stress-induced health breakdown

150 points to 300 points implies about a 50% chance of a major breakdown in the next 2 years

300 points or more raises the odds to about 80%, according to the Holmes -Rahe statistical prediction model

IMPLEMENTING YOUR PLAN

1. **TAKE INVENTORY**
list your stressors
from highest to least

2. **ADDRESS**
elimate, change or respond
differently to stressors

3. **EVALUATE**
tips and techniques you
will use to reduce stress

TAKING ACTION

Step I. Taking Inventory

Identify your stressors by completing the Taking Inventory Form and list your stressors, from the greatest to the least.

Step II- Address the Stressor(s)

After you have identified and listed the stressor. The next step is to choose which method you will use to address the stressor. **E means to eliminate the stressor, C means to change the stressor, and RE means to respond to the stress differently.**

Step III- Your Stress Reliever Plan

The next process is to start working on your Stress Reliever Plan

Step IV – Sample Reliever Plan

See the Sample Reliever Plan as an example to help you

fill out your stress reliever plan

Step IV – Incorporate Stress Free Tips

You may use the tips I've provided in this book to help

you implement your plan or you can use your own tips.

Step V- Review Your Plan

After you have implemented your plan. Review your plan

in 30, 60 or 90 days and see if it's working or if you need

to make adjustments to it. I've included a sample plan as

an example. Change is better if it's done gradually.

Therefore, work on one or two stressors at a time and

then go to the next if you have more. Also, be consistent

and seek professional help or resources if needed.

Remember you are not alone; we can do this together!

TAKING INVENTORY

Step I. Identify Your Stressors:

Write down the things that are causing you to be stressed.
List the stressors according to the highest to the least.
You may not have eight stressors and that's fine. List
each stressor on the line.

1. _____

2. _____

3. _____

4. _____

5. _____

6. _____

7. _____

8. _____

Next Step II –Choose your method to address your stressor(s)

After listing your stressors, go to the next page and complete the form and choose how you will address the stressors by using **E** to eliminate the stressor, **C** to change the stressor, and **RE** to respond to the stress differently.

ADDRESS THE STRESSOR(S)

Your Name:_____

Today's Date:_____

Stressor #1 (Take the stressor you listed and write

it here).

_____

Can you eliminate the stressor? Yes or No

_____ If Yes, how will you go about eliminating

the stressor?

_____

_____

_____

_____

Can you change the stressor that is causing you stress? Yes or No _____ If Yes, what can you change about the stressor?

_____

_____

_____

_____

If you can't eliminate or change the stressor, how can you respond to it differently? If so, what would you do differently?

_____

_____

_____

_____

ADDRESS THE STRESSOR(S)

Your Name:_____

Today's Date:_____

Stressor #2 (Take the stressor you listed and write

it here).

_____

Can you eliminate the stressor? Yes or No

_____ If Yes, how will you go about eliminating

the stressor?

_____

_____

_____

_____

Can you change the stressor that is causing you stress? Yes or No _____ If Yes, what can you change about the stressor?

_____

_____

_____

_____

If you can't eliminate or change the stressor, how can you respond to it differently? If so, what would you do differently?

_____

_____

_____

_____

ADDRESS THE STRESSOR(S)

Your Name:_____

Today's Date:_____

Stressor #3 (Take the stressor you listed and write it here).

_____

Can you eliminate the stressor? Yes or No

_____ If Yes, how will you go about eliminating the stressor?

_____

_____

_____

_____

Can you change the stressor that is causing you stress? Yes or No _____If Yes, what can you change about the stressor?

_____

_____

_____

_____

If you can't eliminate or change the stressor, how can you respond to it differently? If so, what would you do differently?

_____

_____

_____

_____

ADDRESS THE STRESSOR(S)

Your Name:_____

Today's Date:_____

Stressor #4 (Take the stressor you listed and write

it here).

_____

Can you eliminate the stressor? Yes or No

_____ If Yes, how will you go about eliminating

the stressor?

_____

_____

_____

_____

Can you change the stressor that is causing you stress? Yes or No _____ If Yes, what can you change about the stressor?

_____

_____

_____

_____

If you can't eliminate or change the stressor, how can you respond to it differently? If so, what would you do differently?

_____

_____

_____

_____

ADDRESS THE STRESSOR(S)

Your Name:_____

Today's Date:_____

Stressor #5 (Take the stressor you listed and write it here).

_____

Can you eliminate the stressor? Yes or No

_____ If Yes, how will you go about eliminating the stressor?

_____

_____

_____

_____

Can you change the stressor that is causing you

stress? Yes or No _____If Yes, what can you

change about the stressor?

_____

_____

_____

_____

If you can't eliminate or change the stressor,

how can you respond to it differently? If so, what

would you do differently?

_____

_____

_____

_____

ADDRESS THE STRESSOR(S)

Your Name:_____

Today's Date:_____

Stressor #6 (Take the stressor you listed and write it here).

_____

Can you eliminate the stressor? Yes or No

_____ If Yes, how will you go about eliminating the stressor?

_____

_____

_____

_____

Can you change the stressor that is causing you stress? Yes or No _____ If Yes, what can you change about the stressor?

_____

_____

_____

_____

If you can't eliminate or change the stressor, how can you respond to it differently? If so, what would you do differently?

_____

_____

_____

_____

ADDRESS THE STRESSOR(S)

Your Name:_____

Today's Date:_____

Stressor #7 (Take the stressor you listed and write it here).

_____

Can you eliminate the stressor? Yes or No

_____ If Yes, how will you go about eliminating the stressor?

_____

_____

_____

_____

Can you change the stressor that is causing you stress? Yes or No _____ If Yes, what can you change about the stressor?

_____

_____

_____

_____

If you can't eliminate or change the stressor, how can you respond to it differently? If so, what would you do differently?

_____

_____

_____

_____

ADDRESS THE STRESSOR(S)

Your Name:_____

Today's Date:_____

Stressor #8 (Take the stressor you listed and write it here).

_____

Can you eliminate the stressor? Yes or No

_____ If Yes, how will you go about eliminating the stressor?

_____

_____

_____

_____

Can you change the stressor that is causing you stress? Yes or No _____ If Yes, what can you change about the stressor?

_____

_____

_____

_____

If you can't eliminate or change the stressor, how can you respond to it differently? If so, what would you do differently?

_____

_____

_____

_____

75

STRESS

FREE

TIPS

****

TAKE INVENTORY

In order to recognize and relieve stress

let's take a look at what is causing you to

be stressed!

****

1. Identify Your Stressors

Start identifying your stressors by taking inventory of those things that cause you stress. Write down your stressors and begin to work on a plan to either eliminate, change or respond to the stressor differently. Change is most effective if it's done gradually, so don't try to take on too much. Change one stressor at a time, the biggest one first, then move on to the next one. You can use the Stress Reliever Plan to start implementing your plan.

2. Listen to Your Body and Know Your Triggers

Your body is a great indicator of when and why you are feeling stressed. Take a step back and evaluate the stressor (what is causing you stress), so you will know it's trigger and how to respond to it. Sometimes the indicators can be tensed muscles, headaches, irritability, neck tightness, shoulder,

back or chest pain, nausea, digestive problems or

more.

3. Take the Stress Test

The Holmes and Rahe Stress Scale have been used

to determine the amount of stress one experiences in

a year. The scale suggests the higher the score, the

more likely the person is to become ill. You can

search online for the Holmes and Rahe Stress Scale

to rate your stress level or use the one in this book.

```
*************************************
```

CREATING A STRESS-FREE

ENVIRONMENT

Promoting a stress-free environment is

beneficial!

```
*************************************
```

4. Decluttering

Taking the time to declutter your environment is good! It may be time to start donating or getting rid of some old clothes or shoes you don't wear, shredding paper that has been piled up or donating books and magazines that you aren't reading anymore. There's nothing wrong with getting rid of the old to make room for the new. Having an environment that is clean and organized allows good energy to flow. It also allows you to enjoy your space, while promoting relaxation, peace, and harmony without clutter.

5. Use a Do Not Disturb Sign

Posting a Do Not Disturb sign on your bedroom door is ideal for a mother who has young children. Posting a Do Not Disturb Sign will give you an opportunity to do something you like to do, such as watching a good movie, reading one of your favorite magazines, or taking a

relaxing bath without interruptions. Or whatever you like

to do to relax.

6. Use Essential Oils

Using essential oils such as lavender, chamomile,

sandalwood, orange, and lemon can provide a relaxing

environment in your home, car, or workplace. You can

place a few drops in your bath water, diffuser, spray them

in the air, or smell the oil and watch how it will positively

affect your mood.

****

PLAN and PREPARE

You will feel less stressed if you plan and

prepare ahead of time!

****

7. Set a Daily Schedule

Implementing a schedule to balance your personal and professional life is important. Making a daily list in your planner or phone calendar for what needs to be done that day, or the days to come is helpful. Be careful not to book to many appointments or have too many things to do in a day. Don't make your schedule so tight that you don't allow enough time for adjustments.

8. Make a Weekly Chore List

Get your children involved in helping you with chores around the house can help you to have some time for yourself while teaching them good housekeeping and independent skills. Develop chores that are age appropriate and suitable for your child or children.

9. Plan Weekly Menus

Planning weekly menus is helpful. Preparing meals in advance, such as baked spaghetti, lasagna, soups, chilis, casserole dishes, and freezing them for later will save so much time.

10. Prepare the Night Before

Preparing the night before by having breakfast, lunches, and dinners planned and clothes ready for the next day is critical in making your mornings run smoothly. It saves time and energy, and you won't feel as rushed in the mornings.

11. Schedule Family Meetings

Taking time to have family meetings are helpful too. Having these meetings will give opportunities to address family concerns and allow each person to speak and be heard. It's also a great way for families to catch up on each other's lives and feel free to communicate openly.

12. Set Goals

Setting short and long-term goals are helpful. Setting goals allows you to plan and prepare without feeling pressured or overwhelmed by trying to accomplish a task or project in a short period of time. Setting realistic goals can give you the direction you need to set realistic timeline without feeling stressed and rushed. Having a vision board can help with goal setting too.

13. Evaluate Your Finances

Being financially overwhelmed is stressful. Review your finances and plan a course of action to overcome your financial stressors. Becoming proactive about reducing debt and saving for emergencies, vacations, and

retirement will help to ease the burden of financial stress.

14. Set Rituals

Setting relaxation rituals either at the beginning or at the

end of the day are great ways to relieve stress.

Relaxation techniques such as stretching, deep breathing,

or exercising, will help counteract stress.

****

HEALTHY LIVING

Taking care of your body belongs to you!

If you want to get the best out of it, you'll have

to put the best into it.

****

15. Eat Healthy Foods

It is just as important to eat healthy foods as it is to relieve stress. I believe you can't have one without the other. It's noted that stressed individuals are more likely to snack on unhealthy foods, than healthy foods. It's important that we eat for nutrition and not out of being stressed or bored. Eating healthier foods maybe challenging but consuming more raw foods in our diet will fuel our bodies with the proper nutrition that it needs and assist with boosting our immune system. You want to eat foods that fuel your body, instead of foods that are high in sugar, calories, and have no nutritional value.

16. Take Vitamins and Supplements

Taking vitamins such as Vitamin B-12 and Vitamin C are good for stress. To get an extra boost, try a B-complex for energy and to support your nervous system. In addition to that, there is an herb called Ashwagandha that's good for combating stress. Always consult your doctor before adding any vitamins, herbs, or supplements to your regimen.

17. Get Adequate Sleep

It's important that you get the adequate amount of sleep your body requires. Not getting enough sleep will affect your stress level and mood. Studies report that if you don't get enough sleep, you are prone to become more irritable, make poor judgment calls, and have difficulty making decisions. Also, a lack of sleep does not allow your body to rest and heal itself, which can weaken your immune system and make you susceptible to illness.

18. Schedule Medical Exams

It's important to have your annual examinations and screenings for preventive purposes and address any health needs. I see it too often, we put ourselves last and procrastinate going to the doctor which puts our health at risk.

19. Get Rid of Unhealthy Habits

Many times, we can pick up unhealthy habits when we become stressed, such as: drinking alcohol, smoking, overeating and consuming too much sugary, salty and processed foods. Seek to replace unhealthy habits with good habits. Healthy living produces better outcomes. Unhealthy habits could lead to obesity and disease.

20. Enjoy Life

Try your best to live life to the fullest by making healthy choices for your life and your family. Have fun, relax, smile, laugh, and enjoy life! Enjoy being with you and spending time your family and friends.

21. Physical Activity

One of the best ways to relieve stress is doing some type of physical activity for thirty minutes each day. Physical activities, such as walking, dancing, jogging, swimming, bicycling, or other exercises are a great way to keep the body moving and keeping your stress level down, while maintaining a healthy weight.

****

BALANCE

It's not always easy trying to balance the demands of life, but not having balance can make you feel overwhelmed, pressured and stressed.

****

22. *Maintain Balance*

It's important to maintain balance. Balance is defined as equal weights of distribution. We have to ensure that we have balance and maintain balance. When we overextend ourselves in one area, the other areas of our lives become unbalanced. When one area goes lacking or is neglected, it will affect the other areas of your life. The body, soul and spirit need to be in unison with each other.

23. *Slow Down*

It's important that we slow down and take time to smell the roses. Do what you can in a given day. And what you can't do, let it go for another day. Remember the old saying, "Rome wasn't built in a day." We don't want to be so busy rushing that we miss out on enjoying life and enjoying the people God has put in our lives.

24. Balance the Use of Technology

We live in a fast-paced technology driven world. If we are not careful, too much technology, social media, cell phone and Internet usage can be a distraction, especially if we don't know how to balance its use and use it wisely. It's okay to put those devices down, turn it off and take a break from it every now and then.

25. Weigh Your Options

It's wise to consider a matter before you make a big decision or big purchase. Take time to consider the matter before you jump into something. It may sound like a good idea and it may look good, but is it good for you and is the timing right? You don't want to jump into anything too fast that can cause you to feel unbalanced, stressed and you will regret later.

26. Be Mindful of Changes

Don't try to take on too much or have too many major life-changing events within a small period of time. Try to space them out if you can. Too many major life-changing events in a short period of time can increase your stress level and affect your physical and mental health. Some life-changing events cannot be avoided, such as death, illness, or injury. But making major life changing events such as: getting married, going back to college, purchasing a new home, having a baby, or starting a business and etc.., are better for your health and well-being if you can space them out, instead of having too many major life-changing events in a short period of time.

27. Find Hobbies

Finding something you always wanted to do or have an interest in can be the additional thing you may need to bring enjoyment to your life. Starting a hobby can bring you the balance and peace you've been looking for.

28. Complete One Thing at a Time

Multitasking isn't the best option for getting several things done. Focusing on too many things at one time can be stressful. Focus on one thing and finish it before you start something else.

****

ACCEPTANCE

Know that you are unique, special and there

can only be one of you.

****

29. Love Yourself and Be You

It's important to learn to love yourself. Love who you are and who you are becoming. Nobody can be you but you. The more you love yourself and accept who you are, the better you will feel about yourself.

30. Give Up Perfectionism

Don't try to be a perfectionist. Perfectionists tend to be hard on themselves. Trying to be a perfectionist can lead to disappointment and feelings of failure and how you judge and feel about yourself It's okay to let perfectionism go.

31. Let It Go

Whatever you can't fix, don't force it. Just let it go. Maybe it wasn't meant to be, or the timing isn't right. Sometimes we stay in relationships, especially when God has clearly told us to move on. Often times, we are hoping for what we want, instead of what is good for us.

32. Stop Explaining

Sometimes we spend so much time talking and trying to explain ourselves to people who really don't understand who we are. And after the explaining we are left feeling depleted and drained. You don't have to keep explaining yourself, just keep moving and progressing. In the end, they will see the results.

****

SETTING BOUNDARIES

Boundaries are necessary to have in place for

ourselves and others!

****

33. Set Boundaries

Personal boundaries are guidelines, rules, or limits that one establishes for oneself and for others to respect and behave. Many times, we don't set boundaries because we may not know what it means, we don't know we have a voice, or we fear of losing the person or hurting their feelings. Setting boundaries helps us to be empowered and strengthened so that we can stick to our beliefs and morals and not let anyone go against our will or morals. You have to stand for what you believe in. If people have your best interest at heart, they will respect your boundaries and adapt to them. But you have to be clear of what they are and articulate them to others. Often times you have to teach people how to respect and treat you. But it starts with you knowing who you are and what you stand for. *To thine own self be true (William Shakespeare).*

34. Learn to Say No Without Feeling Guilty

Remember you have a voice and a right to say no. Don't allow people to guilt you or pressure you to do something you don't want to do or have the means to do. No is not a bad word.

35. You Can't Change People

Unhealthy relationships can be stressful. Sometimes we can get involved in a relationship believing and hoping we can change an individual. But that person has to want to change. In the meantime, keep working on being the best you can be.

36. Choose Your Battles

Sometimes it's not always a good time to say what's on your mind. It might not be the right time for you to say what you want to say, or the person may not be in a place to hear what you have to say. It may be less stressful to table the conversation for another time.

37. *Know Your Limits*

Making promises and commitments you can't keep can be stressful. Your heart might be in the right place, but finances, time, or your physical or mental well-being may limit you in fulfilling a person's request. It's wise to wait and think before responding too quickly to a person's request. Let the person know you will get back with them instead of committing or making promises you are not able to keep. Only commit to the things that are within your limits and are able to accomplish.

****

EMOTIONAL FREEDOM

In order to have emotional freedom, we have to let go of the past, identify the triggers that affect your emotions and manage your emotions.

****

38. *Forgive Yourself and Others*

Forgiveness is a powerful tool.   In order for you to move forward, you have to forgive those who have hurt you or done you wrong. If you have difficulty forgiving others, and you believe in God, ask Him to come into your heart to help you to forgive. It's just as important that as you forgive others, you forgive yourself too.

39. *Get Rid of Anger*

Sometimes we can carry anger for years due to how we were mistreated, past hurts, the mistakes we've made, and the disappointments and failures we've experienced. Anger could possibly lead to rage, bitterness, and hatred, and it can fester in our hearts and minds if we haven't dealt with the matter. If you are dealing with anger, seek help, and ask God to heal your heart and teach you to let the anger go.

40. Listen Before Reacting

If we are not careful, sometimes our emotions can have us reacting out of anger and frustration when we are in a disagreement with another person. Responding too quickly and harshly out of emotions and anger could possibly affect your stress level, blood pressure, heart rate, your health, and possibly hurt you and the other person as well. You may need to count to ten before you respond, or graciously walk away, or ask the person can you discuss it at another time and when you are in better control of your emotions.

41. Don't Suppress Your Feelings

You have power in your voice. Don't forget to use it. You will feel more empowered when you express your feelings calmly, versus suppressing them. Suppressing your feelings can make you feel irritated, frustrated, and stressed because you are denying how you truly feel. Try expressing your feelings sooner than later, instead of waiting until it builds up and you explode.

42. Let Go of Fear

Fear will keep you in one place and paralyze you from moving forward, but faith will propel you to your destiny. If you let go of fear, faith will take you to places you've never been before.

43. Develop Patience

Being impatient will allow you to make hasty and impulsive decisions without using wisdom. Making hasty and impulsive decisions can lead to regrets and have you feeling stressed about the decision you made. Learning to be patient will allow wisdom to kick in which will produce better outcomes for your life.

44. *Avoid Procrastination*

The best solution to address procrastination is to deal
with what needs to be done. Putting it off, will only
make matters worse. Eventually you will have to address
the matter anyway.

****

HAVE FAITH IN GOD

Continue to put your faith in God and believe

that no matter what it looks like, change will

come

****

45. Have a Relationship with God

If you believe in God and have a relationship with Jesus Christ, He will give you the strength, guidance, courage and peace, you need to become a healthier and balanced individual.

46. Pray

Praying can help to relieve the pressures and stress you may feel and provide you with God's peace during difficult, overwhelming, and stressful times.

47. Stop Worrying

When we take on a spirit of worry, we are doubting that God will work out our situation. Worrying brings on anxiety, fear, tension, stress, and uneasiness, and it doesn't solve anything. It just makes you feel worse. When things are beyond your control, learn to let it go and trust God.

Stay in the present, and don't worry about how it will work out. Have faith in God.

48. Meditate on the Word of God

When we reflect and think on the goodness of God and meditate on His Word, it can offer us hope, peace, joy, and the encouragement we need. It can change the way we think and help us to get focused on the right perspective.

49. Have a Spirit of Gratitude and Thanksgiving

No matter how life may appear to be, learning to be grateful and giving thanks for what you have can provide contentment and peace. Don't focus on what others may have, or where they may be in life. Be thankful and give thanks for what you have, where you are, and where you are going.

****

HAVE FUN

All work and no play is no fun!

Balance your life with fun activities that will

bring enjoyment and laughter to you

****

50. Socialize with Friends

Socializing is good. Going out with a friend or friends is a healthy way to have fun and relax. It can take your mind off things that you might be stressed about.

51. Learn to Laugh More

Sometimes life can have you feeling so uptight and serious that you forget to laugh. Learning to laugh more and taking things lighter is refreshing. If you need help laughing more, watch a funny movie or show to get you laughing again. Laughter is good for the soul.

52. Play Games or Go to an Amusement Park

Playing board or card games or going to an arcade or an amusement park is another way to "let your hair down," and have fun. Be a kid again, run, play and be free.

53. Read a Book or Magazine, Color or Work on a Puzzle

Reading a book or magazine, coloring, or working on a puzzle can help you to relax while taking your mind of your stressors.

****

BE POSITIVE

Surround yourself with positivity instead of

negativity.

****

54. Be Around Positive People

Don't allow negative people to influence your happiness. Surround yourself with positive people who can support your dreams, encourage and believe in you.

55. Keep Dreaming

Never stop dreaming. Keep your dreams alive, and don't let them die. Sometimes dreams have been pushed aside or forgotten. But it doesn't matter how old you are, keep believing and dreaming. Turn your dreams into reality.

56. Use Positive Self-Talk and Affirmations

If you are having negative thoughts, replace them with positive thoughts and affirmations. Using self-affirming words such as "Yes I can," "I'm capable," "I'm worthy and valuable," "I'm beautiful," God loves me, "I'm loved," I am fearfully and wonderfully made are just a few affirmations to begin with.

57. Smile More

Getting into a habit of smiling more will make you feel good and help you to have a positive outlook on life. If you smile, the world may smile back at you. And if they don't, keep smiling anyway.

****

RELAXATION

Free yourself from tension by refreshing the

mind and body.

****

58. Enjoy a Relaxing Bath

Taking a warm bath with your favorite aromatherapy oils is soothing and adding candles to the bathroom will enhance the atmosphere and provide you with a very relaxing experience.

59. Listen to Music

Listening to different genres of music of your choice is a great way to relax and improve your mood.

60. Stretching

Stress can cause your muscles to become tense and tight. But stretching can help to relieve tense muscles. It will also help with circulation and flexibility. Stretching can improve your mood and well-being too.

61. Learn to Relax

Sometimes we may say we are relaxing, but we have difficulty in that area. It's important that we learn to train our minds and bodies to relax and stop our minds from racing and thinking about all the things we need to do, and learn to breathe, exhale, and enjoy the moment we are in.

62. Try Relaxation Exercises

Stretching, walking, and deep breathing are all good stress relievers. They provide relaxation for the mind and body.

63. Enjoying Outdoors

Going to the beach, the mountains, hiking, camping, and traveling are great ways to relax, have fun, and get away from the hustle and bustle of life.

64. Breathe Deeply

Deep breathing can help to relieve stress. It makes you feel calm and relaxed. It provides good blood flow and oxygen to the heart. Sit in a comfortable position with your palms up, eyes closed or open, and shoulders relaxed. Breathe in through your nose while your abdomen and lungs expand and hold for about 5 seconds and the slowly exhale through your mouth while your abdomen flattens. Continue to do this for about ten to fifteen minutes and you will notice the difference and how calm you feel.

65. Listen to Relaxing Sounds

Listening to relaxing sounds, such as ocean waves and nature sounds, can relax your mind.

66. Have a Cup of Hot Tea

Having a cup of hot tea can be relaxing. Teas with lavender, chamomile, lemongrass, spearmint, peppermint, or lemon can be very soothing.

****

SEEK HELP

Don't be afraid to seek help to live a fuller and

productive life

****

67. Seek Wise Counsel

There may be times you may need to talk to someone who can give you wise counsel. Seek wisdom from someone you can trust is a great resource and support system. The wise counselor could be a close friend, relative, pastor, social worker, counselor, or a mental health professional, and etc.

68. Ask for Help and Seek Resources

It may not feel good when you have to ask for help. It can make you feel vulnerable and uncomfortable. But don't let fear or pride stop you from seeking the assistance or resources you need. Getting help will help to relieve the burdens you may be experiencing.

69. Seek Medical Attention

If you are feeling stressed and not feeling well, please

seek medical attention. This book was not written to

replace seeking medical help but to be used for

informational purposes on ways to relieve stress and to

encourage you to seek additional help if needed.

****

HAVE A SUPPORT SYSTEM

We were not created to be isolated or alone! Develop

friendships and relationships with those who love and

support you.

****

70. Have Friends You Can Trust

It's great to have friends you trust. It's important to continue to build healthy relationships with friends who support you, love you, applaud your successes, share your disappointments, encourage you, and can be truthful when you need it.

71. Spend Time with Your Loved Ones

Spending time with your family and friends who love you can bring you the balance you need. Knowing that you are loved and valued is a natural desire we all crave, need and want.

****

TAKING CARE OF YOU

You have a responsibility to your own health

and well-being!

****

72. *Take Mini Vacations*

If you are not in a financial place to take a week or a two-week vacation, start off with a mini vacation. A mini vacation can consist of a weekend or a three-day getaway. Come up with a place you would enjoy going and start planning for your getaway.

73. *Free Your Mind*

A great way to free your mind is to write things down. Don't try to keep everything in your head. Having too much on your mind can clutter your thoughts and can be overwhelming.

74. *Rest*

Many of us have a hard time doing this. We say we are resting, but are we really resting? Resting is defined as ceasing all types of work, movement, or physical activity.

Our bodies need rest so we can be replenished, refreshed, and restored. We shouldn't think that we are so busy that we can't take time out to rest and simply do nothing.

75. Make Time for You

If you haven't already done so, start making time for you. Choose one day a month or a half day a month that's strictly devoted to you. It can be your mental health and wellness day. If money is an issue, find things to do with little cost, or not cost, such as watching a movie, getting a massage at a massage school; getting a manicure, pedicure or facial at a cosmetology school; having a picnic; going to the beach; taking a long walk; going to the park; treating yourself to a special meal; enjoying a relaxing bath with candles and bath oils.

STRESS RELIEVER EXAMPLE

Please see sample below:

Problem/List Stressor: I have a bad habit of arriving to work and to my appointments late. It causes me to become irritated, frustrated, tensed and stressed. Sometimes I end up having headaches and muscle pain in my legs because I am feeling stressed.

(E, C, or R): I plan to change my stressor by getting to work and arriving to my appointments fifteen to thirty minutes ahead of time by leaving earlier planning and preparing the night before by packing my lunch, having my clothes ready and getting gas ahead of time.

30-Day Feedback/Comments: This plan works when I am consistent. I've found out that in order for this plan to work. I need to have an idea of what I will eat for breakfast too, instead of trying to figure it out in the mornings. I will continue to prepare everything at night, including my breakfast, or at least have an idea of what I will eat that morning or bring it to work to eat.

60-Day Feedback/Comments: It's getting better. I'm arriving to work and to my appointments on time or ahead of time which helps to alleviate stress and tension. I'm more aware of my time and I don't cut it so close anymore. I allow extra time for driving, which makes me feel better and less stressed.

90-Day Feedback/Comments: I will continue this plan because it's working, and I don't need to make any adjustments.

Tips I plan on using to relieve stress: I plan on using stress tip #75 by making time for myself and selecting one day a month as a wellness day devoted to me. I also would like to plan on incorporating stress tip #72 by planning a mini vacation.

STRESS RELIEVER PLAN

Today's Date:

Name:

Problem List Stressor #1:

(E, C, or R)

30-Day Feedback/Comments:

60-Day Feedback/Comments:

90-Day Feedback/Comments:

Tips I plan on using to relieve stress:

STRESS RELIEVER PLAN

Today's Date:

Name:

Problem List Stressor #1:

(E, C, or R)

30-Day Feedback/Comments:

60-Day Feedback/Comments:

90-Day Feedback/Comments:

Tips I plan on using to relieve stress:

STRESS RELIEVER PLAN

Today's Date:

Name:

Problem List Stressor #1:

(E, C, or R)

30-Day Feedback/Comments:

60-Day Feedback/Comments:

90-Day Feedback/Comments:

Tips I plan on using to relieve stress:

STRESS RELIEVER PLAN

Today's Date:

Name:

Problem List Stressor #1:

(E, C, or R)

30-Day Feedback/Comments:

60-Day Feedback/Comments:

90-Day Feedback/Comments:

Tips I plan on using to relieve stress:

STRESS RELIEVER PLAN

Today's Date:

Name:

Problem List Stressor #1:

(E, C, or R)

30-Day Feedback/Comments:

60-Day Feedback/Comments:

90-Day Feedback/Comments:

Tips I plan on using to relieve stress:

STRESS RELIEVER PLAN

Today's Date:

Name:

Problem List Stressor #1:

(E, C, or R)

30-Day Feedback/Comments:

60-Day Feedback/Comments:

90-Day Feedback/Comments:

Tips I plan on using to relieve stress:

STRESS RELIEVER PLAN

Today's Date:

Name:

Problem List Stressor #1:

(E, C, or R)

30-Day Feedback/Comments:

60-Day Feedback/Comments:

90-Day Feedback/Comments:

Tips I plan on using to relieve stress:

STRESS RELIEVER PLAN

Today's Date:

Name:

Problem List Stressor #1:

(E, C, or R)

30-Day Feedback/Comments:

60-Day Feedback/Comments:

90-Day Feedback/Comments:

Tips I plan on using to relieve stress:

STRESS RELIEVER PLAN

Today's Date:

Name:

Problem List Stressor #1:

(E, C, or R)

30-Day Feedback/Comments:

60-Day Feedback/Comments:

90-Day Feedback/Comments:

Tips I plan on using to relieve stress:

STRESS QUIZ ANSWERS

1. Is stress avoidable? Yes or <u>No</u> – Stress is not avoidable. We can encounter stressful events throughout the day, but how you respond to the stressful situation can make a difference on how it will affect you.

2. Can stress cause weight loss? <u>Yes</u> or No – Stress can impact an individuals' weight loss or weight gain. In some cases, some people may lose their appetite and not eat, which can cause weight loss.

3. Can too much stress cause belly fat? <u>Yes</u> or No – When the stress hormone called cortisol is released it increases belly fat .

4. Is stress easily diagnosed? The answer is <u>No</u>. It has been reported that stress is the underlying causes to many illness and diseases, which makes it hard for stress to be diagnosed as the root cause.

5. It's reported that 60 percent of doctor's visits are stress-related: True or <u>False</u> – It's reported that 75 percent to 85 percent of doctor's visits are related to stress.

6. Is all stress bad? The answer is <u>No</u>. Examples of good stress are: getting married, purchasing a new home, going back to school, having baby, purchasing a home, starting a business and etc. These are all positive events, but they can come with more responsibility or an adjustment, which can affect your stress level. These events are good, and over time

they will eventually balance themselves out if stress levels are managed

7. Can chronic stress be linked to anxiety or depression?

   True or False – Chronic stress not only affects your physical health, but your mental health too. Chronic stress is linked to anxiety disorder, panic attacks, and depression.

8. Can chronic stress strengthen your immune system?

   True or False – Chronic stress weakens the immune system which makes illness and disease more susceptible to set in.

FINAL THOUGHTS

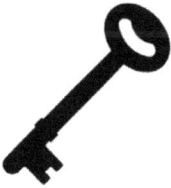

**CONSITENCY
IS KEY**

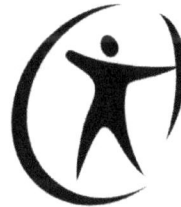

**SEEK
SUPPORT**

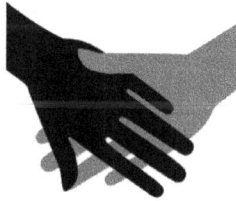

**LISTEN TO
YOUR BODY**

Notes:_____

_____

_____

_____

_____

_____

_____

_____

_____

_____

_____

_____

About the Author

Pamela Wakefield is a writer, author, publisher, minister, entrepreneur and survivor of chronic stress. Pamela is passionate about writing and writes from her heart. She writes to inspire, inform and bring about change in the lives of her readers.

Pamela's vision is that her books will promote wholeness and healing to the mind, body and soul that will bring forth change, healing and deliverance to individuals, families, and communities.

Pamela is a mother and grandmother who resides in Raleigh, North Carolina. For more information about Pamela, and/or to purchase her books, products, services, or products you can visit her website at www.pamelawakefield.com or you can email her at info@pamelawakefield.com